Peripheral T-Cell Lymphoma:
Fast Focus Study Guide

JT Thomas, MD

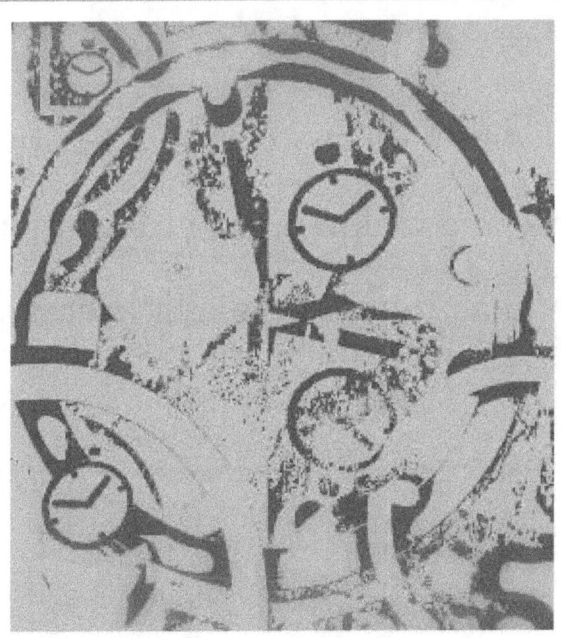

Acknowledgements

I dedicate this book to my beautiful wife and children, who I love more than all the water in all the oceans and all the seas.

CONTENTS

- This book is written to help the reader further understand the Peripheral T-Cell Lymphoma.

- This book is written in a simple and easy to read format designed for medical students, residents and physicians who are preparing for boards.

- This book simplifies a complicated medical issue so you will remember the important details.

- You will not get caught up in the minutia. Just the facts are found in this book.

- This Fast Focus Study Guide will provide you with a practical review of the key information you need to know.

- Buy this book now if you want this quick and concise information

This book is going to review the peripheral T-cell lymphomas. These are a diverse group of uncommon and sometimes aggressive diseases.

T-cell lymphomas can be a group of diseases that are easy to confuse. I like to divide this group of diseases into 4 big categories. These categories are Cutaneous T-cell lymphoma, Extranodal T-cell lymphoma, Nodal T-cell Lymphoma, and Leukemic T-cell Lymphoma.

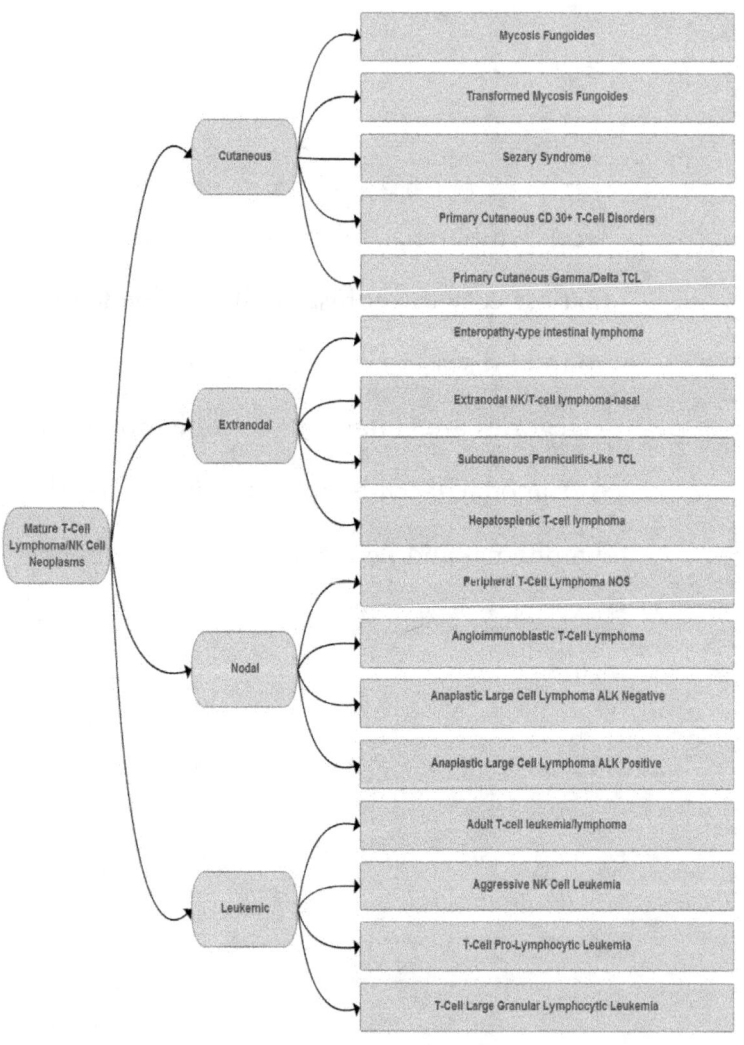

Let us have a look at each of these categories starting with the cutaneous T-cell lymphomas.

The cutaneous T-cell lymphomas are generally a group of indolent lymphomas with the exception of Transformed Mycoses Fungoides which behaves in a more aggressive fashion.

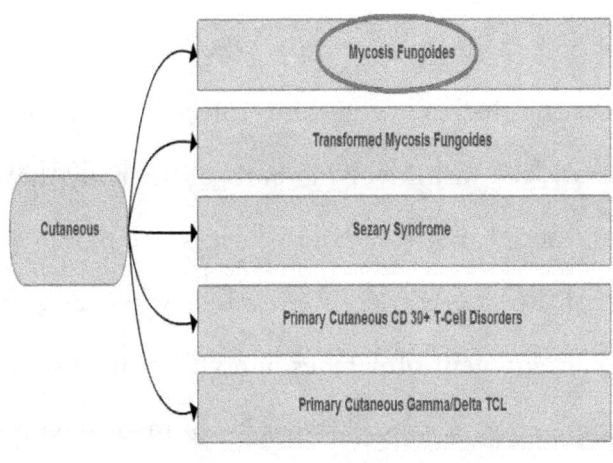

Cutaneous T-cell lymphomas: Mycosis Fungoides

Mycosis fungoides is a type of cutaneous T cell Lymphoma made up of mature T-helper lymphocyte cells that originates in the skin. It typically presents as a scaly, red rash involving parts of the body that are not necessarily sun exposed. It is commonly a disease of the elderly that progresses slowly over years with development of patches of erythematous skin and plaques. In advanced stages it can involve lymph nodes.

Cutaneous T-cell lymphomas: Mycosis Fungoides

Mycosis fungoides is the most type of common cutaneous T-cell lymphoma. It is rare in individuals under 50 years of age. If the lymphoma develops into soft tissue tumors and becomes systemic and the prognosis is poor.

Cutaneous T-cell lymphomas: Mycosis Fungoides

Mycosis Fungoides is characterized by skin infiltration of CD4 + malignant lymphocytes with nuclei that have characteristic cerebroid morphology.

Cutaneous T-cell lymphomas: Mycosis Fungoides

Mycosis fungoides can be treated with local therapy or systemic treatment. Local mycosis fungoides therapy can include topical therapy such as steroids, retinoids, topical chemotherapy, and psoralen-enhanced light therapy. Additional local therapy options include radiation, intralesional steroids, and surgical removal. Systemic therapy includes oral retinoids, recombinant IFN-α, monoclonal antibodies, single-agent chemotherapy, histone deacetylase inhibitors, and extracorporeal photopheresis.

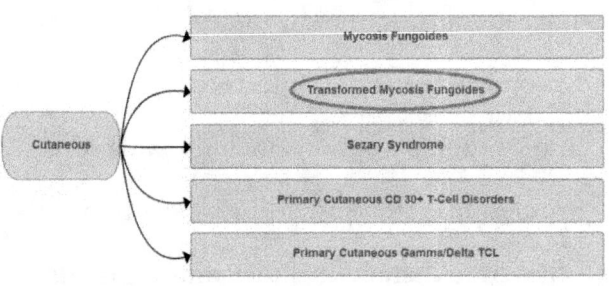

Cutaneous T-cell lymphomas: Transformed Mycosis Fungoides

Mycosis fungoides can transform into a more aggressive disease characterized as a large T-cell lymphoma. This transformed mycosis fungoides is characterized by the presence of more than 25% of large cells on biopsy of an mycosis fungoides skin lesion.

Cutaneous T-cell lymphomas: Transformed Mycosis Fungoides

When transformation occurs, the median time from diagnosis of MF to transformation was 6.5 years. Mean survival from transformation to death was 22 months.

Cutaneous T-cell lymphomas: Transformed Mycosis Fungoides

The median survival of mycosis fungiodes is 163 months, but the median survival in patients with transformed mycosis fungoides is 37 months.

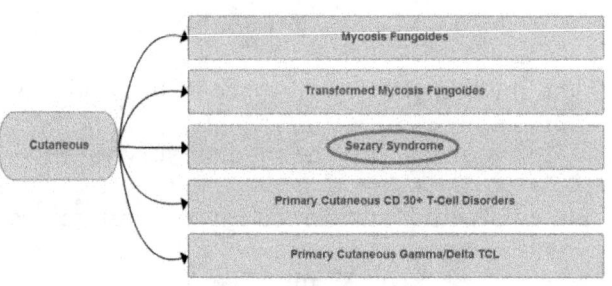

Cutaneous T-cell lymphomas: Sézary syndrome

Sézary syndrome is a T-cell disorder characterized by both skin and peripheral blood involvement.

Cutaneous T-cell lymphomas: Sézary syndrome

Sézary syndrome is associated with pruritis and erythema of the skin sometimes with desquamation.

Cutaneous T-cell lymphomas: Sézary syndrome

Sézary syndrome is the second most common form of cutaneous T-cell lymphoma after mycosis fungoides.

Cutaneous T-cell lymphomas: Sézary syndrome

Sézary syndrome can be treated with systemic monotherapies including extracorporeal photopheresis, interferon alpha, bexarotene, low-dose methotrexate, denileukin diftitox (plus corticosteroid). Useful combination therapies include Interferon with PUVA or topical nitrogen mustard; methotrexate with topical nitrogen mustard; bexarotene with PUVA; immunomodulators such as ECP, interferon alfa or gamma, bexarotene (singly or in combination) with total skin electron beam radiation.

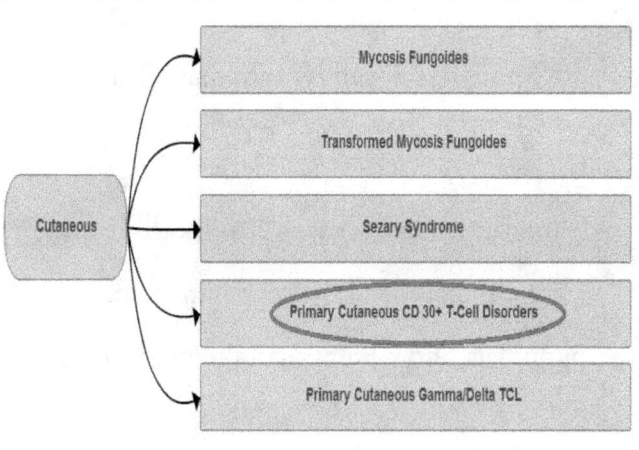

Cutaneous T-cell lymphomas: Primary Cutaneous CD 30+ T-Cell Disorders

Primary Cutaneous CD 30+ T-cell disorders are characterized by both lymphomatoid papulosis and primary cutaneous anaplastic large cell lymphoma.

Cutaneous T-cell lymphomas: Primary Cutaneous CD 30+ T-Cell Disorders

Lymphomatoid papulosis is a rare disease in the category of cutaneous T-cell lymphoma and more specifically it is a type of primary putaneous CD 30+ T-cell disorders.

Cutaneous T-cell lymphomas: Primary Cutaneous CD 30+ T-Cell Disorders

Lymphomatoid papulosis is more common in females. It presents as a self healing subcutaneous nodule that develops on the face, trunk, extremities, and genitals. They often will disappear in 3-12 weeks only to recur again.

Cutaneous T-cell lymphomas: Primary Cutaneous CD 30+ T-Cell Disorders

Cutaneous anaplastic large cell lymphoma is a type of primary cutaneous CD 30+ T-cell disorder. It is composed of large T-cells that appear anaplastic and pleomorphic. More than 75% of these cells are positive for CD30.

Cutaneous T-cell lymphomas: Primary Cutaneous CD 30+ T-Cell Disorders

Cutaneous anaplastic large cell lymphoma is more common in women. It commonly seen in HIV+ patients.

<u>Cutaneous T-cell lymphomas: Primary Cutaneous CD 30+ T-Cell Disorders</u>

Cutaneous anaplastic large cell lymphoma presents as ulcerated nodules and papules with skin involvement. It is often multifocal and only rarely will have lymph node involvement.

Cutaneous T-cell lymphomas: Primary Cutaneous CD 30+ T-Cell Disorders

In nodal anaplastic T-Cell lymphoma, ALK negative disease is associated with a worse prognosis. The cutaneous form of anaplastic T-Cell lymphoma is typically ALK negative, however the prognosis is usually good.

Cutaneous T-cell lymphomas: Primary Cutaneous CD 30+ T-Cell Disorders

Primary cutaneous CD 30+ T-cell disorders include both lymphomatoid papulosis and cutaneous anaplastic T-cell lymphoma. If characteristic skin lesions do not resolve, then low dose methotrexate or radiotherapy can be used. Combination chemotherapy should not be used unless the patient develops extracutaneous disease.

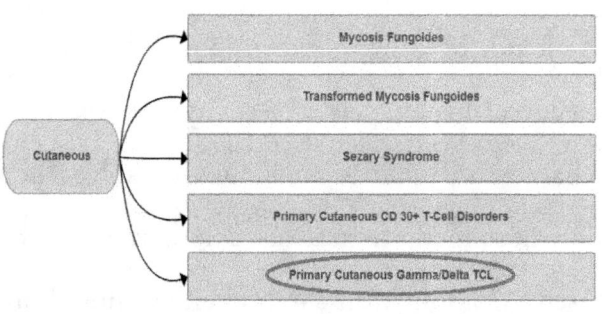

Cutaneous

- Mycosis Fungoides
- Transformed Mycosis Fungoides
- Sezary Syndrome
- Primary Cutaneous CD 30+ T-Cell Disorders
- Primary Cutaneous Gamma/Delta TCL

Cutaneous T-cell lymphomas: Primary Cutaneous Gamma-Delta T-cell Lymphoma

Primary cutaneous gamma-delta T-cell lymphoma originates from activated mature gamma-delta T cells with a cytotoxic phenotype is a rare T-cell lymphoproliferative disease.

Cutaneous T-cell lymphomas: Primary Cutaneous Gamma-Delta T-cell Lymphoma

Primary cutaneous T-cell lymphoma is a rare disorder estimated that accounts for approximately 1% of cutaneous T-cell lymphomas. This disease often presents as ulcerated plaques and/or nodules.

Cutaneous T-cell lymphomas: Primary Cutaneous Gamma-Delta T-cell Lymphoma

This disease is characterized by a bad prognosis associated with a poor response to chemotherapy.

Cutaneous T-cell lymphomas: Primary Cutaneous Gamma-Delta T-cell Lymphoma

Primary cutaneous gamma-delta T-cell lymphoma is often treated with CHOP chemotherapy sometimes combined with prednisone, psoralen, ultraviolet irradiation, and external beam radiation.

We have reviewed the cutaneous T-cell lymphomas. Let us now have a look at the extranodal T-cell lymphomas. This group of diseases are among the peripheral T-cell lymphomas. There are 4 types of extranodal T-cell lymphomas. These include the Enteropathy-type intestinal lymphoma, Extranodal NK/T-cell lymphoma-nasal, Subcutaneous Panniculitis-Like TCL, and Hepatosplenic T-cell lymphomas.

Extranodal T-cell lymphomas as a group are aggressive diseases with a relatively poor prognosis. Let us start with the Extranodal T-Cell Lymphoma: Enteropathy-type Intestinal Lymphoma.

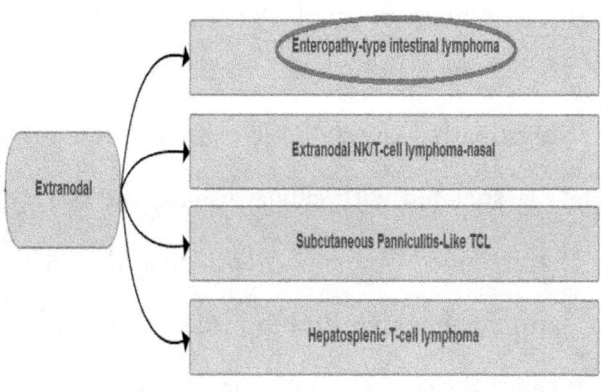

Extranodal T-Cell Lymphoma: Enteropathy-type Intestinal Lymphoma

Enteropathy-associated T-cell lymphoma is associated with celiac disease and is characterized by neoplastic intraepithelial T lymphocytes that develop in patients with celiac disease who are unresponsive to a gluten-free diet.

Extranodal T-Cell Lymphoma: Enteropathy-type Intestinal Lymphoma

Enteropathy-associated T-cell lymphoma can sometimes be treated with surgery to remove the damaged small intestine. Chemotherapy with a CHOP based regimen can be used.

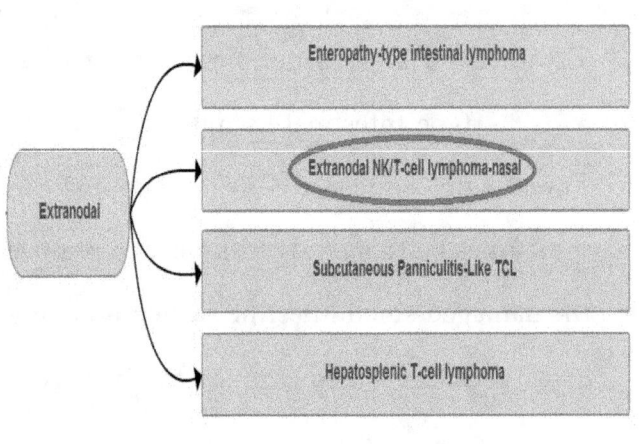

Extranodal

- Enteropathy-type intestinal lymphoma
- Extranodal NK/T-cell lymphoma-nasal
- Subcutaneous Panniculitis-Like TCL
- Hepatosplenic T-cell lymphoma

Extranodal T-Cell Lymphoma: Extranodal NK/T-cell lymphoma-nasal

Extranodal NK/T-cell lymphoma, nasal type, is a rare disease more common in Central America, South America and Asia.

Extranodal T-Cell Lymphoma: Extranodal NK/T-cell lymphoma-nasal

Extranodal NK/T-cell lymphoma, nasal type, can be characterized by malignant T cells or malignant natural killer cells.

Extranodal T-Cell Lymphoma: Extranodal NK/T-cell lymphoma-nasal

Symptoms can include facial swelling, nasal discharge or bleeding, and nasal congestion or blockage. Extranodal NK/T-cell lymphoma, nasal type, typically effects the nose, nasal passages, or paranasal sinuses.

Extranodal T-Cell Lymphoma: Extranodal NK/T-cell lymphoma-nasal

This disease is usually associated with Epstein-Barr virus. A high level of circulating EBV is associated with more extensive disease and worse prognosis.

Extranodal T-Cell Lymphoma: Extranodal NK/T-cell lymphoma-nasal

Early stage extranodal NK/T-cell lymphoma-nasal is treated with a combination of chemotherapy and involved-field radiotherapy (dose > 50 Gy). Late-stage disease is treated with chemotherapy alone. Regimens containing L-asparaginase and gemcitabine might be better than CHOP but are associated with increased toxicity.

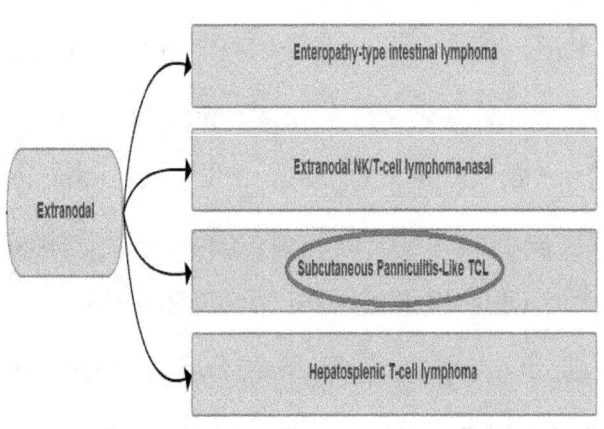

Extranodal T-Cell Lymphoma: Subcutaneous Panniculitis-Like TCL

Subcutaneous panniculitis-like T-cell lymphoma is a rare form of extranodal lymphoma characterized by multiple nodular deep subcutaneous erythematous lesions that can be quite large. Sometimes patients will develop plaques involving the legs, arms, trunk and face.   Usually there is no lymph node involvement, but lymph nodes can be involved

Extranodal T-Cell Lymphoma: Subcutaneous Panniculitis-Like TCL

The nodules that characterize this disease can have spontaneous resolution initially but they subsequently will return to involve the same or different areas.

Extranodal T-Cell Lymphoma: Subcutaneous Panniculitis-Like TCL

This disease has a median age of 43 years. It is more common in women. Patients often have pancytopenia.

Extranodal T-Cell Lymphoma: Subcutaneous Panniculitis-Like TCL

This disease is associated with poor prognosis related to a severe hemophagocytosis with a median survival is usually < 2 years.

Extranodal T-Cell Lymphoma: Subcutaneous Panniculitis-Like TCL

Combination chemotherapy with a CHOP based regimens are typically given to treat subcutaneous panniculitis T-cell lymphoma. External beam radiation has been proven effective in certain clinical situations.

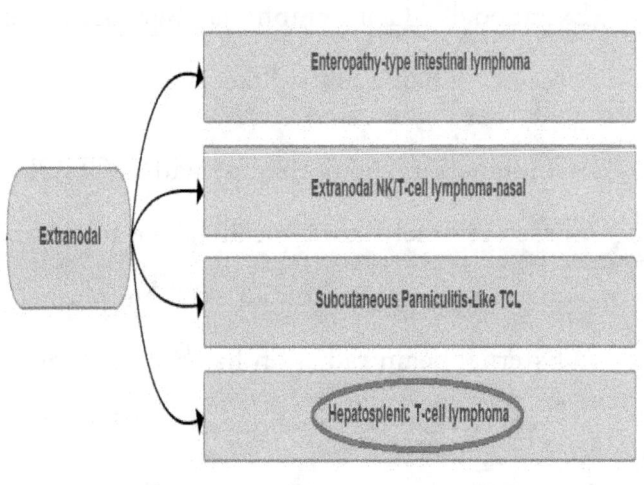

Extranodal T-Cell Lymphoma: Hepatosplenic T-cell Lymphoma

This disease is associated with poor prognosis related to a severe hemophagocytosis with a median survival is usually < 2 years.

Extranodal T-Cell Lymphoma: Hepatosplenic T-cell Lymphoma

Combination chemotherapy with a CHOP based regimens are typically given to treat Hepatosplenic T-Cell Lymphoma

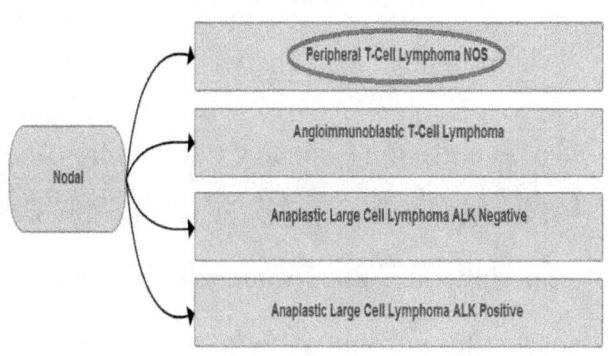

Nodal

Peripheral T-Cell Lymphoma NOS

Angioimmunoblastic T-Cell Lymphoma

Anaplastic Large Cell Lymphoma ALK Negative

Anaplastic Large Cell Lymphoma ALK Positive

Nodal T-Cell Lymphoma: Peripheral T-cell Lymphoma Not Otherwise Specified

This is a group of nodal T-cell lymphomas that do not fit into any of the other subtypes of peripheral T-cell lymphoma. This is the most common subtype of peripheral T-cell lymphoma.

Nodal T-Cell Lymphoma: Peripheral T-cell Lymphoma Not Otherwise Specified

This disease has a median age of 60 years. It is more common in men than women. Patients commonly present with widespread lymphadenopathy. These cancers are often CD4+, CD8–, and CD30+.

Nodal T-Cell Lymphoma: Peripheral T-cell Lymphoma Not Otherwise Specified

Patients often develop fevers, night sweats, and weight loss. Other symptoms can include eosinophilia, pruritis or hemophagocytic syndrome. >60% of patients present with stage IV disease at diagnosis.

Nodal T-Cell Lymphoma: Peripheral T-cell Lymphoma Not Otherwise Specified

Peripheral T-cell Lymphoma Not Otherwise Specified can involve the liver, bone marrow, gastrointestinal tract, and skin.

Nodal T-Cell Lymphoma: Peripheral T-cell Lymphoma Not Otherwise Specified

This group of diseases are characterized by aggressive behavior and poor prognosis. Treatment generally includes systemic chemotherapy with CHOP. Despite chemotherapy, the 5 year disease free survival is 25%.

Nodal T-Cell Lymphoma: Peripheral T-cell Lymphoma Not Otherwise Specified

Peripheral T-cell lymphoma NOS is treated with systemic chemotherapy with treatments including CHOEP, CHOP, fludarabine, pentostatin, and gemcitabine. Other treatment options include radiation, alemtuzumab, and romidepsin.

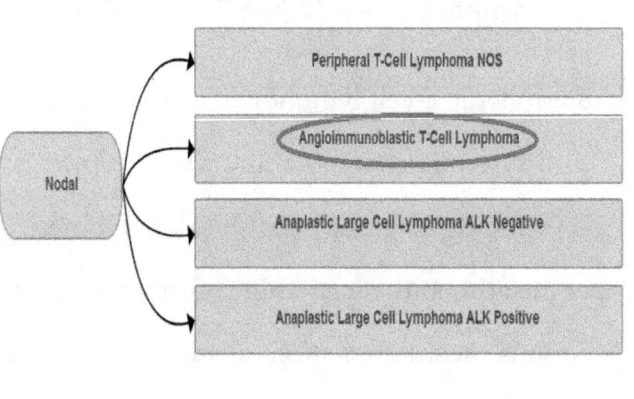

Nodal T-Cell Lymphoma:

Angioimmunoblastic T-cell lymphoma

Angioimmunoblastic T-cell lymphoma accounts for 1-2% of all cases of NHL and 15 — 20% of T-cell Lymphomas. This group of diseases are characterized by aggressive behavior and poor prognosis.

Nodal T-Cell Lymphoma:

Angioimmunoblastic T-cell lymphoma

Angioimmunoblastic T-Cell Lymphoma is the second most common T-cell lymphoma. Symptoms often include pruritis, arthritis, and skin rash. This cancer is associated with EBV and Epstein-Barr virus (EBV) genomes are can be detected of in large B cells within the infiltrate.

Nodal T-Cell Lymphoma:

Angioimmunoblastic T-cell lymphoma

Angioimmunoblastic T-Cell Lymphoma has the phenotype of a follicular T-helper cells. These cells express CD10 CXCL13 and PD1CD10, CXCL13, and PD-1. Patients often have a monoclonal or polyclonal gammopathy. It is not unusual for patients to present with stage III or stage IV disease associated with organomegaly, pleural effusions, and B symptoms.

Nodal T-Cell Lymphoma:
Angioimmunoblastic T-cell lymphoma

Angioimmunoblastic T-cell lymphoma is associated with a poor prognosis. The reported 5-year OS of approximately 30% and median survival of 3 years.

Nodal T-Cell Lymphoma:
Angioimmunoblastic T-cell lymphoma

Angioimmunoblastic T-Cell Lymphoma can relapse as diffuse large cell B cell non-hodgkins lymphoma.

Nodal T-Cell Lymphoma:

Angioimmunoblastic T-cell lymphoma

The autoimmune symptoms of this disease can be treated with steroids. This cancer is often treated with combination chemotherapy such as CHOP.

Nodal T-Cell Lymphoma:
Angioimmunoblastic T-cell lymphoma

Angioimmunoblastic T-cell lymphoma is typically treated with a CHOP based chemotherapy regimen.

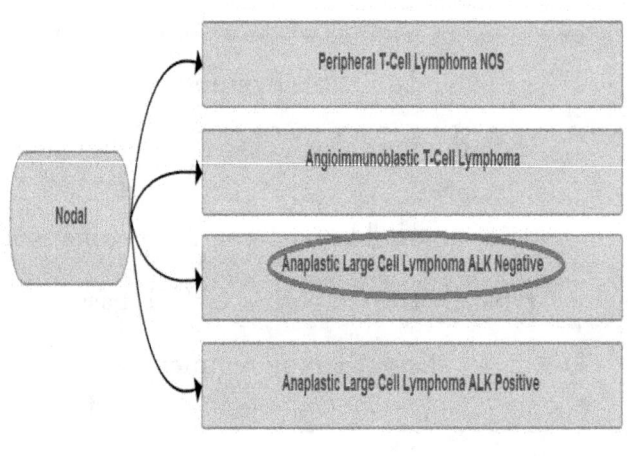

Nodal T-Cell Lymphoma: Anaplastic Large Cell Lymphoma ALK Negative

Anaplastic large-cell lymphoma is a nodal T-cell lymphoma. This peripheral T-cell lymphoma involves the lymph nodes but often has extranodal involvement with involvement of the skin, liver, bone, and brain.

Nodal T-Cell Lymphoma: Anaplastic Large Cell Lymphoma ALK Negative

Anaplastic large-cell lymphoma always expresses CD 30 and other T-cell lymphomas variably express CD 30.

Nodal T-Cell Lymphoma: Anaplastic Large Cell Lymphoma ALK Negative

Anaplastic large cell lymphoma is characterized by large T-cells that expresses CD3 and CD30. Anaplastic large cell lymphoma can be divided into ALK negative disease and ALK positive disease. ALK expression is due to a fusion gene produced by the t(2;5) translocation that juxtaposes the genes for ALK and nucleophosmin.

Nodal T-Cell Lymphoma: Anaplastic Large Cell Lymphoma ALK Negative

ALK negative disease is often seen in older patients and is associated with a poor prognosis which often progresses during chemotherapy or relapses soon after the completion of treatment.

Nodal T-Cell Lymphoma: Anaplastic Large Cell Lymphoma ALK Negative

Patients with ALK negative anaplastic large cell lymphoma who also have the DUSP22 rearrangements have a better prognosis.

Nodal T-Cell Lymphoma: Anaplastic Large Cell Lymphoma ALK Negative

Anaplastic Large Cell Lymphoma is treated with CHOP based chemotherapy.

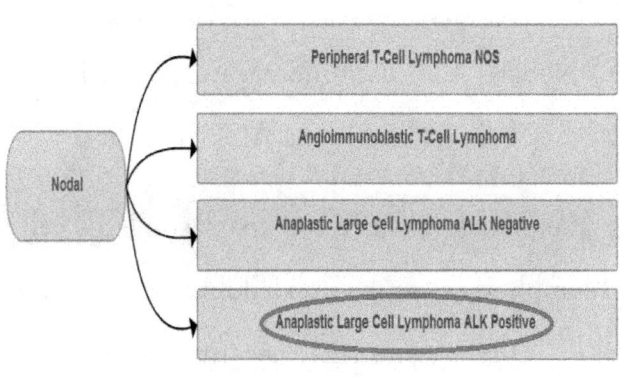

Nodal T-Cell Lymphoma: Anaplastic Large Cell Lymphoma ALK Positive

As noted above, T-cell anaplastic large-cell lymphomas can be divided into ALK positive disease and ALK negative disease.

Nodal T-Cell Lymphoma: Anaplastic Large Cell Lymphoma ALK Positive

ALCL ALK-positive disease is characterized by the nucleophosmin (NPM)-ALK fusion protein, generated by the t(2;5)(p23;35) translocation.

Nodal T-Cell Lymphoma: Anaplastic Large Cell Lymphoma ALK Positive

ALK positive anaplastic large cell lymphoma can be stratified based on international prognostic index. If the IPI is 0-1 then the disease behaves less aggressively. If the IPI is greater than 1 the disease has a worse prognosis.

Nodal T-Cell Lymphoma: Anaplastic Large Cell Lymphoma ALK Positive

Anaplastic Large Cell Lymphoma usually responds well to chemotherapy, so it often has a good prognosis is treated with CHOP based chemotherapy.

Now let us talk about the Leukemic T-Cell Lymphomas. These include adult T-cell leukemia/lymphoma, aggressive NK cell leukemia, T-cell pro-lymphocytic leukemia and the T-cell large granular lymphocytic leukemia.

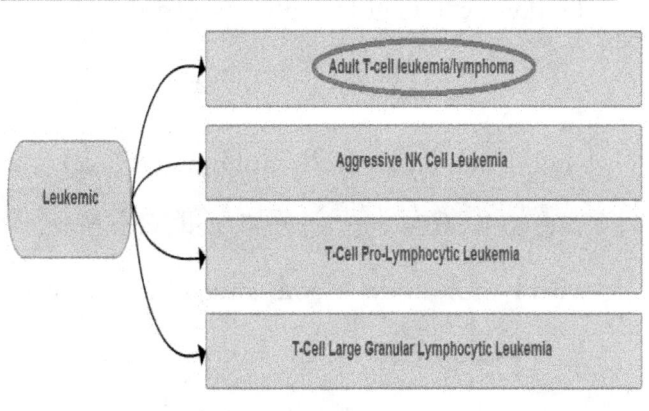

Leukemic T-Cell Lymphoma: Adult T-Cell Leukemia/Lymphoma

Adult T-cell leukemia/lymphoma (ATLL) is a rare and often aggressive T-cell lymphoma with lymph node, blood, and skin infection associated with the human T-cell lymphotropic virus type 1 (HTLV-1).

Leukemic T-Cell Lymphoma: Adult T-Cell Leukemia/Lymphoma

Human T-cell lymphotropic virus is in the Retroviridae family and was the first retrovirus discovered. It is an RNA virus that uses reverse transcriptase to produce DNA from RNA. HTLV affects T lymphocytes.

Leukemic T-Cell Lymphoma: Adult T-Cell Leukemia/Lymphoma

Less than 5% of individuals with HTLV-1 will develop adult T-cell leukemia/lymphoma.

Leukemic T-Cell Lymphoma: Adult T-Cell Leukemia/Lymphoma

HTLV1 associated adult T-cell leukemia will often present with hypercalcemia.

Nodal T-Cell Lymphoma: Adult T-Cell Leukemia/Lymphoma

Adult T-cell leukemia/lymphoma can be characterized by the immunophenotype:

Immunophenotype: CD3 +, CD4 +, CD5 +, CD7-, CD25 +

Nodal T-Cell Lymphoma: Adult T-Cell Leukemia/Lymphoma

Adult T-cell leukemia/lymphoma can be separated into: acute, lymphomatous, chronic and smoldering.

Leukemic T-Cell Lymphoma: Adult T-Cell Leukemia/Lymphoma

Acute and lymphoma type adult T-cell leukemia/lymphoma typically have a poor prognosis.

Leukemic T-Cell Lymphoma: Adult T-Cell Leukemia/Lymphoma

The prognostic factors include performance status, lactate dehydrogenase, age, number of involved lesions and hypercalcemia. Other factors include Ki-67 expression, p53 mutations, p15INK4B/p16INK4A abnormalities and overexpression of interferon regulatory factor 4.

Leukemic T-Cell Lymphoma: Adult T-Cell Leukemia/Lymphoma

Adult T-Cell Leukemia/Lymphoma is typically treated with the antiviral AZT in combination with a CHOP based chemotherapy regimen.

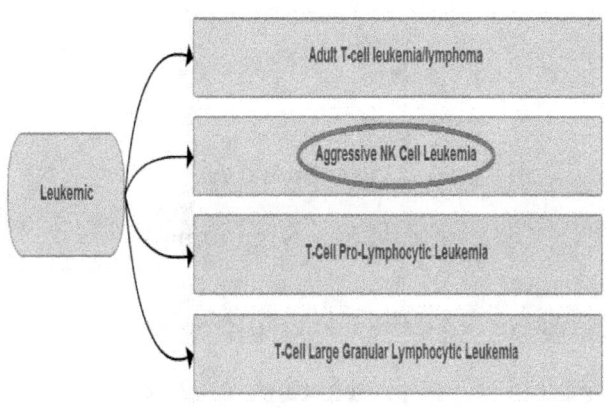

Leukemic T-Cell Lymphoma: Aggressive NK-cell leukemia/lymphoma

Aggressive NK-cell leukemia/lymphoma with a median age of presentation at 42 years old. Patients present with rapidly progressive symptoms associated with weight loss, jaundice and fever.

Leukemic T-Cell Lymphoma: Aggressive NK-cell leukemia/lymphoma

Aggressive NK-cell leukemia/lymphoma is a very aggressive disease characterized by skin infiltration, lymphadenopathy and hepatosplenomegaly. Patients often have anemia and thrombocytopenia associated with hemophagocytosis.

Leukemic T-Cell Lymphoma: Aggressive NK-cell leukemia/lymphoma

Aggressive NK-cell leukemia/lymphoma typically has circulating cancer cells. DIC with abnormal liver tests is commonly seen. This disease is extremely aggressive and many people only live a period of weeks after diagnosis.

Leukemic T-Cell Lymphoma: Aggressive NK-cell leukemia/lymphoma

Aggressive NK-cell leukemia/lymphoma is often treated with a regimen know as SMILE. This regimen consists of S – Solumedrol; M-Methotrexate; I-Ifosfamide; L-Asparaginase; and E-Etoposide.

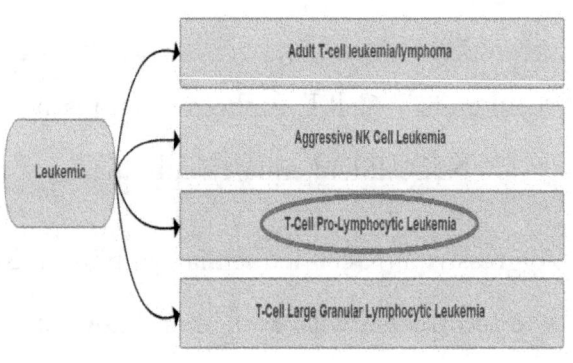

Leukemic T-Cell Lymphoma: T-Cell Prolymphocytic Leukemia

T-cell-prolymphocytic leukemia is a rare T-cell leukemia with a poor prognosis. The disease is characterized by skin, liver, and spleen involvement.

Leukemic T-Cell Lymphoma: T-Cell Prolymphocytic Leukemia

Patients often present with a lymphocyte count > 100,000 associated with skin involvement, splenomegaly, and diffuse lymphadenopathy. HTLV-1 testing will be negative and there will be no evidence of a monoclonal gammopathy.

Leukemic T-Cell Lymphoma: T-Cell Prolymphocytic Leukemia

T-cell prolymphocytic leukemia has a poor prognosis and is often resistant to chemotherapy. Most patients need immediate treatment. Treatment options include alemtuzumab, CHOP, purine analogues. Stem cell transplant is indicated in selected patients who respond to initial treatment.

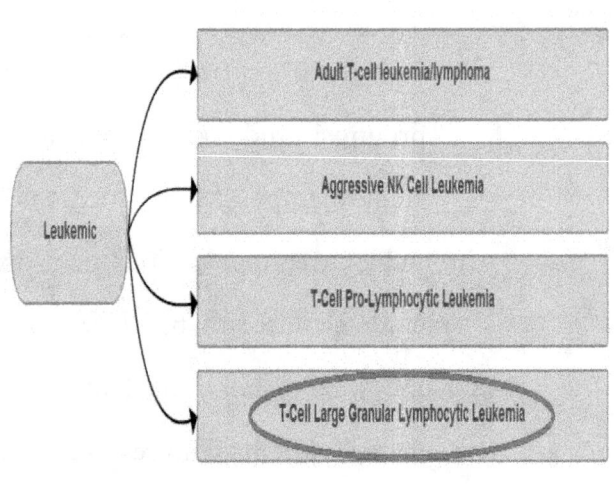

Leukemic T-Cell Lymphoma: Large Granular Lymphocytic Leukemia

Large granular lymphocytic leukemia is an often indolent disease that is characterized by neutropenia associated with lymphocytosis of large granular lymphocytes that have CD8. Many of these lymphocytes also express CD3 although some of these cells will have NK expression.

Leukemic T-Cell Lymphoma: Large Granular Lymphocytic Leukemia

About 80% of these patients will have neutropenia and 45% of these patients will have severe neutropenia.

Leukemic T-Cell Lymphoma: Large Granular Lymphocytic Leukemia

T-cell large granular lymphocytic leukemia has a median age of 60 years and accounts for 85% of diagnosis in Western countries.

Leukemic T-Cell Lymphoma: Large Granular Lymphocytic Leukemia

Autoimmune disorders such as Sjögren's syndrome rheumatoid arthritis, systemic lupus erythematosus, and Hashimoto's thyroiditis commonly are seen in patients with T-cell large granular lymphocytic leukemia.

Leukemic T-Cell Lymphoma: Large Granular Lymphocytic Leukemia

Active surveillance is undertaken if the patients are asymptomatic. Many patients will eventually become symptomatic. Treatment should be considered if the patient develops recurrent infections, severe neutropenia, symptomatic anemic, symptomatic thrombocytopenia, symptomatic splenomegaly or the onset of systemic symptoms.

Leukemic T-Cell Lymphoma: Large Granular Lymphocytic Leukemia

There are many possible treatments. Probably the most commonly used treatment is oral low-dose methotrexate administered weekly. About 50% of patients who are treated with methotrexate will develop a complete response. Additional treatment options include cyclophosphamide and cyclosporine A. Sometimes the patient will have improvement of symptoms without resolution of neutropenia. Responses can take several months and at least 4 months of treatment is required before you can say the treatment has failed.

Peripheral T-Cell Lymphomas

This concludes the summary of peripheral T-Cell lymphomas. We reviewed the four subcategories of peripheral T-cell lymphomas (cutaneous, extranodal, nodal, and leukemic). We reviewed 17 different diseases that fall into these categories. As a group these are aggressive lymphomas. The cutaneous T-cell lymphomas tend to be less aggressive and the extranodal, nodal, and leukemic tend to be more aggressive (with the exception of large granular lymphocytic leukemia).

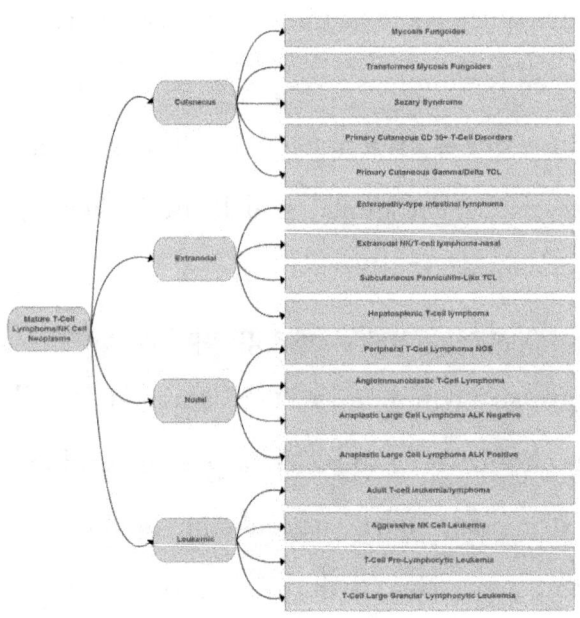

Now let us review some of the new

medications that are available.

Brentuximab

Brentuximab vedotin is an anti-CD30 monoclonal antibody conjugate.

Brentuximab

The most common adverse events associated with brentuximab vedotin include peripheral neuropathy and fatigue.

Bexarotene

Bexarotene is a third generation retinoid approved for the treatment for cutaneous T-cell lymphoma.

Bexarotene

Bexarotene side effects include rash, pruritis, leukopenia, headache, weakness, central hypothyroidism, hypercholesterolaemia and hyperlipidemia.

Vorinostat

Vorinostat is a histone deacetylases inhibitor (HDAC) used for the treatment of cutaneous T cell lymphoma approved for second line treatment or recurrent disease.

Vorinostat

Vorinostat has several potential side effects including fatigue, diarrhea, nausea, hyperglycemia, and thrombocytopenia. Vorinostat is also associated with DVT and PE.

Romidepsin

Romidepsin is a histone deacetylases inhibitor (HDAC) used for the treatment of cutaneous T cell lymphoma approved for second line treatment or recurrent disease was approved for the treatment of CTCL.

Romidepsin

Romidepsin side effects include nausea, vomiting, fatigue, infection, loss of appetite, anemia, thrombocytopenia, and leukopenia, electrolyte abnormalities and cardiac arrhythmias.

Pralatrexate

Pralatrexate is an antifolate antimetabolite approved for treatment of peripheral T-cell lymphoma that stops or slows critical enzymes involved in DNA synthesis triggering cell death.

Pralatrexate

Pralatrexate is associated with leukopenia, thrombocytopenia, hepatic toxicity, tumor lysis, skin reactions. Pralatrexate associated oral stomatitis is improved if treated with supplemental b12 and folate.

This concludes Diagnosis of the Bleeding Patient:

Fast Focus Study Guide

Search Amazon Kindle books to find other study

guides written by

JT Thomas, MD

Internal Medicine Study Guide

Hematology Study Guide

Medical Oncology Study Guide

Cardiology Study Guide

Multiple Myeloma Study Guide

Differential Diagnosis Study Guide

Rheumatology Study Guide

Cancer Study Guide